Table of Contents

ISBN: 9798329333275

Introduction

There's only one real reason you should eat. And that is because you are hungry.

The other reasons are just excuses.

Why are you hungry?

Hunger is the body's way of telling us that it's low in energy. It has to replenish that energy. Otherwise, it will have a food crisis and go into survival mode. What that could mean is that it will try to get energy from its reserves, which may be something you would like if you are trying to cut the fat cells out.

But the other thing that the body will do is slow down organ functions so that it does not use up too much energy. So, the next time you take in some food, the body will try to store more of it to make sure that it will have enough reserve in case you decide to ignore or postpone satisfying its cries for more energy again.

Just because you feel hungry, though, does not mean you will eat whatever you want. You also have to consciously supply what your body needs. We're not going into the details of that. Suffice it to say that you should provide your body with the recommended daily allowance of necessary nutrients that's appropriate for your age, sex, body type and health conditions. And not much more.

Now, you have to realize that there are other triggers for the hunger response apart from the depletion of physical energy. The feeling of being hungry could mean you are experiencing some stressors that are affecting your emotional or psychological state.

Emotional eating is when you respond to a certain feeling with food. Ever heard of comfort foods? That could be an example of emotional eating. When you had just gone through a tough day or had a major fight with your partner, you might feel a strong urge to grab two or three pieces of your favorite double chocolate coated donut.

It could also be emotional eating when you insist that you need to celebrate an accomplishment (however small) with a double cheeseburger treat. You could be using food as a way to increase or maintain your euphoria from winning.

Eating as a response to an emotion or feeling may not actually make you hungry but your mind will send out the signal anyway that you need to eat something. This disturbs your body's natural patterns and may cause you to make unhealthy food choices, the ones that don't help you nutritionally or even sabotage your body's health. For instance, you may feel you deserve a second piece of that giant cupcake because, what the heck. Cupcake makes you feel happier than your ex ever did! Sugar alert!

Then there are eating disorders which are about a person's psychological condition. There is such a thing as binge eating. This is an uncontrolled intake of food, sometimes food items that the person would normally avoid. This may be followed by an episode of purging as is the case with bulimia patients. Or it may result in a person becoming overweight or obese.

Persons with eating disorders have to be medically treated and the person concerned may need psychological therapy. Just imposing a diet on such a person will not help, and it may even be more harmful to force them to eat a certain way. However, a diet may be part of their therapy.

So why go on a diet?

There is also only one reason to do this. And that is for health reasons.

We may be more specific here. Your doctor told you that you need to lose (or gain) weight. Or you may need to create a diet plan because of a certain medical condition such as diabetes or hyperacidity. Or you may need to increase your intake of certain nutrients (ladies, think iron).

Whatever your reason for going into a diet may be, it should be about you not another person. I mean you are not going on a diet because your husband or wife will love you more if you lost weight. You should not follow a diet plan simply because a lot of people around you are into it but you don't really need to.

Not all diets are suitable for everyone. This is not a one size fits all affair. Take care to ensure that the diet is right for you. Consult your doctor, especially if you have known medical conditions.

Also, I strongly recommend that you don't do this on your own. Have an accountability partner who will help you stay on the diet or help you realize when you are overdoing it (yes that is possible).

That said let me tell you why I think the following chapters will help you succeed in your efforts to diet.

During my annual physical exam, the doctor noted that I was overweight and borderline diabetic. He recommended I lose weight, at least 12 pounds (ideally closer to 20 he said) or he will have to recommend I take maintenance meds. He didn't give me a timeline but I didn't like the idea of meds on a regular basis. So, I took him seriously.

I did not follow a strict diet program. I didn't really diet at all. I did lower my food intake. And I tried the techniques I talk about here.

Well, it worked. My weight went down. Two physicals later, I was cleared. No maintenance meds, thank you.

Three years after I was told to get my weight down, I've been able to keep it down. The drop was slow but steady. And I went way within the acceptable weight for my height and age.

The slow drop in weight was important because it helped me avoid a problem that most dieters experience when they exit a diet plan. The gains they got from their diet quickly dissipate once they resume their old eating patterns. And if they go back to the diet, it becomes more difficult to get the same good results. I call this the rebound effect.

Because my weight dropped slowly, my body was able to adjust and not react as if there was a food crisis. This allowed me to sustain the weight loss and keep the gains I got.

So, if you want to try what helped me, read on.

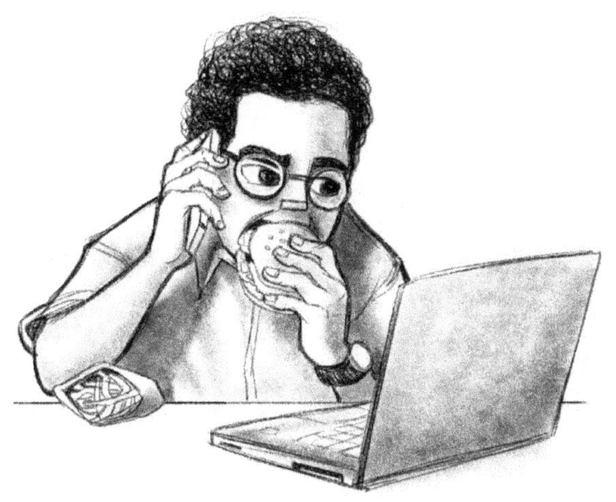

Stop Multitasking

Imagine this. You are watching a movie on your home theater system. It's one you've really been wanting to watch for a while. You just happen to be alone on movie night because for some reason, everybody else has their own thing.

On the table beside you is a tub of popcorn and a glass of your favorite non-alcoholic drink. The movie is engrossing. The popcorn is cooked just right. And of course, an occasional sip is satisfying.

Without looking, you dip your hand into the bucket of popcorn to get a few more. You are surprised to realize that the tub is empty. You've eaten all the popcorn.

Now, tell me this. At what point in the movie did you munch the last piece of popcorn?

You probably can't answer that. What you might be able to say is what scene you were watching when you realized that there was no more popcorn in the tub. And when the realization hit you, you checked the tub to confirm that there was indeed no popcorn left in it.

In that split second, you missed a couple of crucial lines of dialog. Or you may have been surprised that the scene had switched when you looked back at the screen and you aren't sure how they got there.

You were **multitasking**.

The problem with multitasking is you can't focus on two tasks at the same time. Shifting your focus means you lose your concentration on the other task. That's of course, natural. That's how the brain works. Humans are not wired to be multitaskers. But we do it anyway.

In today's fast paced lifestyle, you probably do this; multitask while eating. You munch a breakfast sandwich while you drive to the office (you'll wash the car on Saturday). You work through lunch to get that project done while you down a salad (mind crumbs don't go into the keyboard). You're checking your social media while breezing through your dinner (ooh so many likes, eh?).

You're trying to do two things at the same time. How's the food? Taste good? Did you realize you did not use the dressing that came with the salad?

Researchers have established that there are connections between how attentive we are to the process of eating and how we manage our weight. Distracted eaters tend to go hungry quicker while those who eat mindfully tend to not gain unwanted weight. Eating in a focused way have also been shown to help binge eaters manage their tendencies so that they actually have less incidents of binging.

There's a time for everything. And you have to make time for everything you need to do. Including eating. If you don't focus on the task of feeding yourself, there's a possibility that you either overeat or not eat enough.

Eating too much is, of course a no-no when you are on a diet. That's why you have to watch every morsel that you put into your mouth. But when you're multitasking, you may not realize it's time to stop eating. Like the last popcorn that you did not know was gone, you might find yourself eating beyond when you're supposed to because you were focused on doing something else.

You can prevent this with proper preparation. That is, make sure you set out just the right amount of food before you start eating and doing something else. That may help if you don't have other distractions.

On the other hand, even if you prepare the right amount of food, you might find that you will not be able to finish eating all of it. When you work while having lunch (or have lunch while you continue to work), the work may take so much of your attention that you don't get to eat your entire intended lunch. You may put what's left of the food aside and decide to eat later.

Well, there goes your diet. And, yeah, even if you did not eat more than you should, you still disturb the progress of your diet because you did not eat what you should have.

You'll probably get hungry earlier than usual and give in just to stay standing. Maybe you'll get back to that salad. Or maybe not. In any case, according to your diet, that should not be how you do it. And there goes your diet again.

So focus on just one thing at a time. Whether it's eating, working, reading email or what have you, you'll be more productive and more satisfied if you tackle each task one at a time.

There are other ways that you actually multitask while eating.

You prepare the next spoonful while you're still chewing something.

You talk while you are getting a portion of food from the service plate.

Obviously, the keyword here is "while". In both examples, your focus is not on what you are doing with the food. And in both examples, the tendency is for you to take in too much food.

When you are preparing a spoonful while still chewing, you will most likely put that spoonful in your mouth the moment you swallow what's currently in there. This does not give your system a chance to process the food and tell the brain that it has had enough, you're full.

But even if you're already full, there's now something else in your mouth and your digestive system will still process that. You've overeaten. Maybe you'll say it's just one mouthful but, hey you're on a diet remember?

When you are talking while placing food on your plate, you're not really looking at the size of the portion you are getting. And most probably you will eat what's on your plate however much that is.

I'm not saying there should be no conversation at the dinner table (we'll talk about this later). But again, when you're talking, just talk and focus on the other person. This is just being polite.

When you're getting food to your plate, make sure you're watching your portions. Make sure you're getting the right amounts and the right pieces.

When I was a kid, my dad laid down the law. At mealtime, you are either eating at the dinner table or doing something else away from it without taking food. No TV dinners for him even if he loved TV. Mealtime was all about eating and bonding with the family. TV time was for personal entertainment.

Nowadays, the rule should be no gadgets at the dinner table. Your social media can **wait**. You don't have to jump every time a notification comes in. Give your phone a little rest and yourself a short break from all the noise on the net. The point is to focus on one thing at a time.

The big benefit of focusing while eating is that you know exactly how much you are getting into your body. If you are on a diet, you get to watch your intake precisely. That helps you stay on track and that's exactly what this is all about.

It also gives your digestive system the environment to do its work properly. When you're not focusing on your eating, the brain and the rest of the body might mix up their cues. You won't know when you're full and would want to eat more because your brain did not give the signal to stop putting food in your mouth.

Your digestive system might not be able to absorb all the nutrients it should be getting from the food because stuff to digest is coming in too rapidly and they have to be pushed out quickly to make room for more.

So remember, no more TV dinners. Or you can have TV dinners without the television in front of you. Or your phone for that matter. Keep these distractions away from your eating area.

Now, what if a call comes in? Depending on the perceived urgency (juicy tidbits can wait), you can either answer it or drop the call and send the person a quick SMS that you're busy at the moment. Or you can ignore it totally and inform the person of your reason after you finish eating.

What about ambient sounds? Music is fine, there's some use to it when you're eating (more on this later). However, I suggest you stick to instrumental music and not familiar songs that might make you want to sing along. Focus on your food, not the background sounds.

It's a fast paced life we live nowadays. That's why it's important to set aside time for the things you need to do and do right.

Eating is one of those things.

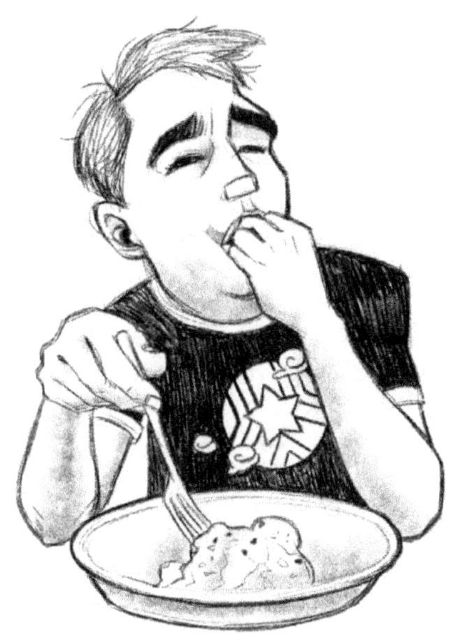

Take It Slowly

Some people eat this way

Chomp-ch-chew-ch-swallo-chomp-ch-chew-ch-swallo-chomp . . .

That is, they chew their food in a hurry and swallow after just a few times masticating. Sometimes, the food they were chewing hasn't even reached the throat area and they've already taken another bite or another spoonful.

Digestion starts in the mouth. Saliva serves to soften the food and the teeth work to cut the food up into small bits so that they easily pass through the digestive path.

The smaller bits also make it easier for enzymes and bacteria along the path to extract the necessary nutrients.

Now, if you rush the food in your mouth just to get over the meal as quickly as possible, you actually make it harder for your body to process the food. Besides, if your food is not broken down well enough by your pearly whites, there's a chance it will stick somewhere and block the food passages. One possible result is choking.

That's because there's a passage at the back of the mouth where both the air we breathe and the food we eat goes through. The body has its own mechanism to control the passage so food goes into the esophagus and air goes to the bronchial system. If a chunk of food that's not well-chewed gets stuck there, air passage may be blocked and the person can experience choking.

So start your digestion right by chewing your food well. Do it this way.

bite-chew—chew—chew—. . .—chew—chew—
swallow

There's another reason why you need to take it slowly, and it has a lot to do with your diet. You see, it's not actually the amount of food you eat that's used by the body to establish that you've eaten enough. It's what the system is able to extract from the food you eat.

If your food is not well-digested, your body will not realize that it has taken in enough food and will not give the signal that you are already full. Thus, you will continue to consume food. And, hey, you're on a diet, remember? But you still feel hungry, so what are you going to do?

So, reserve enough time for your meals. Make time to eat and go slow on your food. Eat comfortably too. Really sit down and eat.

Yes, that's also important, your position while eating. It's not a good idea to eat while walking (hey, that's multitasking) or even standing up. Research has shown that standing and moving about tends to make you eat more or delay the body's realization that it has consumed enough food. That's because your eating position is causing you to consume more energy which the meal also has to replenish.

Besides, being seated for a meal makes your brain believe that you are actually eating a meal and not just having a snack. The benefit here is that your brain will know that you will not need to eat for a longer period because you have consumed a full meal already.

When we eat, all five senses are at work, not just the sense of taste. The process of eating begins with our eyes--the plating will entice you into the meal. Then your nose will raise or drop your expectations about the taste of the dishes in front of you. The sense of touch notices the texture of the food we are eating, whether it's your fingers or your tongue that's touching the food. When we are chewing, our ears sense the crunchiness or other sounds that happen inside the mouth.

Proof of this is what happens when people are asked to identify food items while they are deprived of sight and smell. Most people usually get them wrong. Hmm, this could be a fun party game, don't you think?

There is also such a thing as mindful eating. That is, being conscious of what you are eating and how you eat.

While I was going through mindfulness training, we were asked to experience this. During lunch, we were told to eat alone on the roof deck of the building. No communicating, just you and your food. Afterwards, we discussed what we ate. Being mindful of the food requires concentration and time to savor the food.

It was also during that experience that I realized how to focus on eating slowly and better digesting my food. You see, not far from the building was a construction site. On that particular day, one worker decided to pound some steel during the lunch hour. I was not able to see what he was doing but I could hear his hammer. He was doing it in a rhythmic pattern.

As I ate, I timed my chewing with his pounding. That made me more conscious of what I was eating. It also made me chew my food better.

To help you understand how to do slow rhythmic chewing, try this exercise. When you eat, play the Bobby McFerrin song **Don't Worry Be Happy**. All you have to do is chew food only every time he snaps his fingers. And then finish a stanza of the song before swallowing.

Here are a few more titles you might want to try for this exercise.

> The Longest Time by Billy Joel
> Boy From New York City by Manhattan Transfer
> One More Night by Maroon 5
> Count On Me by Bruno Mars

You don't have to do this at every meal. In fact you shouldn't. But doing it once will give you a good idea of how it feels to eat slowly. Just remember the experience at your next meal. I'm pretty certain you'll find yourself eating at a slower pace and maybe getting to eat less while still being fully satisfied at the end of your meal.

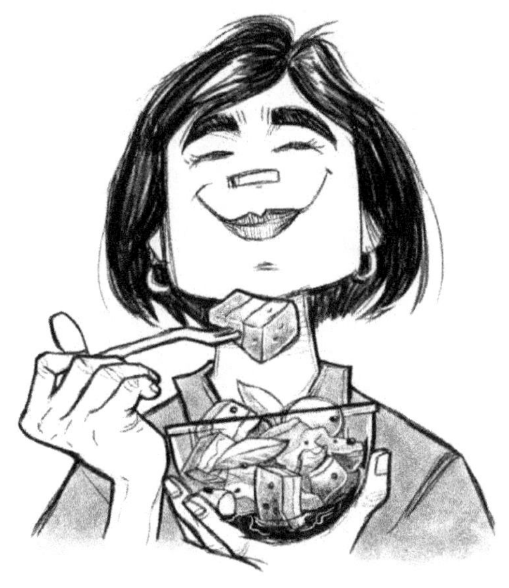

Enjoy Your Meal

I do volunteer work for our church organization where I
and other volunteers report just a few days a week.
One fine day, while we were at the office and enjoying
some snacks, a colleague blurted out, "How come
these chips taste better here than they do at home?"

Sounds silly, doesn't it? How can a certain mass
produced food item like potato chips in a bag taste
differently when eaten in different places?

Actually, there's a reason for that. At home during snack
time on weekdays, she's usually alone. Her husband is
probably out seeing clients for their business or
transacting with the bank. There, she eats the chips by
herself. She'll probably rush through the bag and leave

the table as soon as she can. That is, if she even eats them at the table.

In the office, she eats at a much slower pace, savoring each piece. Between mouthfuls, she joins the conversation and the laughter. The fun that we have while taking a break from work enhances the taste of the potato chips. It's really all in the mind.

If you're on a diet, chances are the food items you have to eat are not the ones you would choose to eat. These are not really what would make your meals enjoyable. It's even possible you are forced to eat some stuff you absolutely hate. But since you are trying to accomplish something, you tolerate them. Well, you will but only until you reach your goal and end the diet, right?

Or the items in your diet plan may actually be things you normally like to eat. However, the idea that your consumption is strictly regulated by your diet may be putting a damper on your enjoyment.

Like my coworker, it's possible to make your mealtimes more enjoyable and, thus make the food tastier. As she discovered, eating with company improved the taste of her chips.

In fact, this whole affair of dieting can be more fun and enjoyable. And that will definitely help you succeed, no matter what your diet program is or what your goals are in doing this.

From the get go, dieting will at least be more tolerable if you have a diet buddy. Find someone in your circle to go through this time with you. They may have their own reasons for dieting, and they may even be on a different program. But having someone you can talk with about what you are going through will make the ordeal of dieting more bearable.

Your buddy could also help keep you on track as you both check on each other's progress. You can set up milestones together, signposts along the way where you can mark accomplishments. You may want to eat one meal together every day, or if that's not possible, weekly dates with each other so you can share good news, 'fess up and encourage each other.

Whether you eat with someone or diet alone, the ambience of your eating space is important. Make sure the atmosphere is relaxing and stress free. For you, it will mean meal time will be enjoyable. For your digestive system, it will mean it can smoothly process what you are eating.

That's why distractions like TV programs and social media notifications are not encouraged during meal times. They actually add to your stress levels apart from taking your focus from your meal.

Ambience is important during a meal. Music is a good way to create that ambience. The right kind can help you enjoy your meal.

Think about it. Fine dining restos and fast food joints are all eating places but their ambient sounds are different. Restaurants tend to play soft jazzy music with a slow tempo that sounds relaxing. This is meant to make you sit down and stay longer. And hopefully, order some more food.

Meanwhile fast foods often play pop and rock tunes that could sometimes dominate the place. The sound is chosen to move things more quickly. They want you and the food to move, and fast.

For meal times, mid-tempo classical instrumental music is recommended. Avoid music with vocals and familiar lyrics so you will be less likely to be tempted to sing along and transfer your focus to the song. With instrumental music played softly, you can leave them in the background and let them work subtly on your brain. You enjoy them but they are less distracting.

The reason for the tempo is obvious. Too fast and you might be tempted to eat just as fast. Too slow and the music might make you feel lethargic which means you might not enjoy what you are doing because you'd rather doze off.

Volume is also important here. You don't want the music to be so loud that it will jar your senses. We eat with all our senses so you want yours to be sensitive to the food experience. So keep it low. Think elevator music.

Then there's plating. Remember that your visual sense is one of the first ones that encounter your food. A meal that is presented well will raise your desire to partake of it, even the food items that you don't particularly relish.

Arrange the food so that they look good on the plate. Imagine that you are serving yourself in some fine dining establishment. You first take the role of the kitchen worker who assembles the food (it's not always the chef). Then you switch roles and become the client who will enjoy this gastronomic masterpiece.

As you sit down to eat, take note of the colors and the texture of the food. Notice how vivid the colors of those crisp vegetables are. Check out the different ingredients that you can distinctly see on that granola bar. Go ahead and laugh at how funny the dish looks that you would want to get it out of your sight as soon as possible. By eating it of course.

Then, as you slowly consume each mouthful, try to distinguish the taste that each ingredient contributes to the dish. Where are the bits of pepper in there? Relish every bit, whether it's savory or sweet. Look for the umami taste in each bite. Hmm. After this, you might be able to get a job as a food taster, eh?

You can do these things whether you are eating alone or you have company at the table. When there's company, the time would be more enjoyable if there was a lively conversation going on. If you aren't really fond of the items on your diet plan, having these conversations would certainly help you tolerate the food you have to eat.

Remember though that you are not supposed to multitask. That is, you don't talk while you have food in your mouth. Chew the food well then swallow. Only then can you respond to the other person. And then, when you finish talking, that's when you work on your next mouthful.

Sure, this will make the conversation flow at a slower pace and will seem to lose its dynamic. Hey, you're here to eat together so go ahead and eat. It will also slow down your speed of taking in food giving your system time enough to determine and give the signal when you have had enough to eat. It will also allow you to notice that signal more easily.

Go ahead and give these ideas a try. It may take some getting used to but it will definitely help you succeed.

Enjoy your meal.

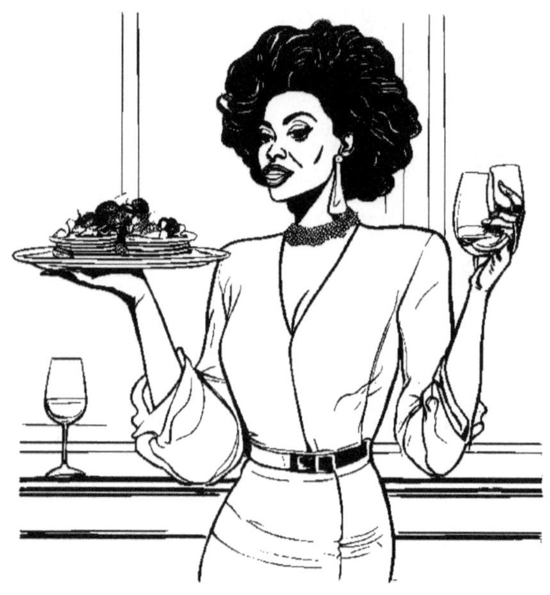

Put It Down

You know this scene. You may have even been part of it.

Two people at a cocktail party are having an animated conversation. They are holding a glass in one hand and hors d'oeuvre in the other. They get so excited about what they are talking about that they start gesturing. Suddenly someone interrupts them to let them know that one of their drinks has spilled.

Or how about this scene?

You are sitting at a table in a fast-food munching on your burger with fries on the side. You hold the burger in one hand and use the other hand to pick one of the fries. You are about to put the fry in your mouth when up walks an old mate who introduces his companion. You want to shake hands with your new acquaintance but what about the food in your hands?

What are you supposed to put down while eating? A lot, actually.

First of all, you have to make sure that what you're eating is going down properly. It's not getting stuck between your teeth, that's going to get you a toothache later especially if you can't brush properly soon after.

It's not going to obstruct your air passage because of its size when you don't chew it thoroughly. You will not choke because of the big pieces. Plus, it will pass through your digestive track smoothly.

It's not going to go back up because you've overwhelmed the bacteria in your stomach and acid is being sent back to where it came from. It won't cause anything like constipation or something similar (Are you eating while reading this, sorry but you're multitasking). Well, that's why it's important to start digesting food in the mouth.

There are other things that would be advisable for you to put down while eating. Think about what you keep in your hands during the meal. Put them down.

Put down your utensils between uses. Forks, knives, spoons all belong on the plate when you are not using them to get food into your mouth. Leave them there while you chew up what's in your mouth at the moment. That's simply good etiquette.

Put down the sandwich and the pizza between bites. You don't have to be holding them the whole time. Do the same with the corn cob, the watermelon, the apple or whatever it is that you are taking bites from.

Put down the tea cup or coffee mug or wine glass or whatever liquid container is there after you take a sip or drink. This is a safety issue. You would not want to unintentionally spill the liquid on yourself or somebody else who just happens to be too close. Even if you have a napkin in front of you, it still would not look good and you know you will be uncomfortable.

Speaking of napkin, put it down on your lap. It's not a bib and you're not a baby anyway.

Seriously, keep your hands free and clean. You might have to use them to shake hands or give someone your business card. Surely you don't want a potential business partner to touch something greasy or moist.

When your sandwich and utensils are not in your hands, you don't rush the next mouthful into your system. If you are holding your pizza, chances are you will take the next bite upon swallowing the previous one. But if it's not in your hands, there will be that extra effort and time to take it up again and have another bite.

Since you're on a diet, putting down the things you eat with or drink from allows you the time to consider the next step in your meal. Should you have some more of that salad? Does your program allow you to take more than two sips of wine? It sure is expensive but what about your diet, eh?

You will probably find this the most difficult of the steps I'm giving you. It feels so natural to be connected with the food using your hands. You want to be ready to continue with your meal so you keep the "weapons" in your hands.

That's the point, actually. Bear in mind that our aim is to keep you from straying from your diet program. Putting down the things you would normally be holding while consuming a meal will help you to take a break and evaluate whether or not you are on track or straying from your program.

So, keep your hands free while your mind works out your next step.

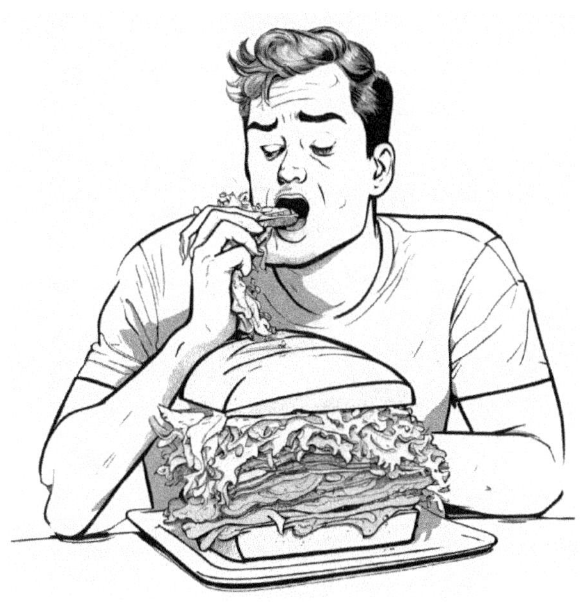

Size Does Matter

I once noticed a new eating place in the mall. Outside, they posted pictures of plated pork chops (their specialty). The chops looked huge because they covered most of the plate. By adding the garnish and the side, the plate was almost entirely covered. Curious, I went in and ordered some food.

The serving did justice to the picture. The plate was full. The food was arranged exactly as it was in the posted picture.

Then I noticed something. The plate was not a regular size dinner plate. Its diameter was about two or three centimeters shorter than what you might expect. So the chops were not exactly as large as you would have imagined from the picture.

Hey, I'm pretty sure you've heard this before. Eat smaller portions. Just eat less (instead of going on a formal diet program). That's actually the main thing I did.

But based on my own experience, it's not just about how big you choose to make the portions.

Let's start with that--food portioning. If you're following a diet program you're probably already watching your portion sizes. You measure out your cereal, count the inches of meat, use a graduated cylinder for your liquids, etc. Good for you if you are able to sustain this.

Now, what will you do after you complete your program? Are you still going to pour your juices into that graduated cylinder before putting it in your glass to drink? Will you keep that ruler around to make sure your meat and vegetable cuts are just the right size. Is that weighing scale staying put in the kitchen? You're no longer on a diet so probably not.

But to sustain what you have gained (or lost) while you were on a diet, you have to avoid going back to your old eating habits. And here is where portion size really matters. You may be able to eat whatever you like, especially those that were prohibited by your program. However, that does not mean you will binge on them because you missed them.

The keyword here is control. You don't have to be as rigorous as while you were on that diet. But you do want to at least maintain the gains you got from following your strict diet. Heck, you might even want to do better.

But you'd also like to have your "normal" life back.

Here are a few things you can try. Even if you are not on a diet or never went on a strict diet program (like me), you might find these things useful so that you don't grow horizontally or should I say rotund.

When ordering pizza, ask the store to cut it into 10 or 12 slices instead of the usual 8. That would mean each slice is smaller than the usual. Then eat the number of slices you would normally consume. Congratulations, you've just eaten a smaller portion of pizza.

Of course, there will be left overs and of course you can eat them later but not just now. You can save them for your next meal. This trick of smaller slices also works with cakes and pies.

With pizza or a burger or a fruit or a sandwich, try this. Place the usual size in your mouth but don't bite just yet. Pull your food out just a tiny bit then take a bite. That would mean you have taken a smaller bite than you normally do. Remember to chew well before swallowing and put it down until you have swallowed what's in your mouth. You can also try this with a granola bar or a chocolate bar or even your favorite donut.

Wait, you're still eating the same burger size. Well, if you got yourself a smaller portion then, no you won't even if you finish the whole thing. Plus, if you attempt to count the number of bites you take, you might find that you'll be biting more or less the same number of times whether or not you take a big or small bite.

Say you're eating something like macaroni or veggies. Before you place it inside your mouth, just go ahead and remove one or two pieces of macaroni from your fork. Better yet, when getting the Mac from a serving plate or bowl, resist the temptation to get that second or third scoop. This also works with cereal or ice cream.

When you buy snacks like potato chips or popcorn, opt for the smaller containers. They are not as cost effective but they do help you lessen unhealthy food intakes. Eat slowly and never look back at the counter.

By taking smaller food portions, you will end up eating less. Your brain will give the signal that you have had enough to eat even if you eat less. What will happen is the digestive system will send a message to the brain that it's handling enough food bits already. Then the brain will inform the whole body that you're full.

There are health benefits to eating smaller portions. Your body is less likely to be overwhelmed by too much glucose in the blood, which may happen if you eat a lot of carbohydrates. You avoid the risk of heartburn, which happens when your stomach is processing a lot of food and your good bacteria produce a lot of acid way beyond the normal level. You also lower the possibility of constipation, which could happen when your intestines are not able to properly handle some big chunks of food.

Consuming food portions that are smaller than the usual amount you eat may seem difficult. Admittedly, it does take a little practice before you get it. That's why other elements of your meal should also be adjusted to enable you to eat less.

When I began working on dropping my weight, I shifted to a smaller plate for my meals. This helped because it still felt like I was filling my plate with the usual food but actually I was eating less. While, you're at it, you might also want to use smaller bowls and smaller size silverware (not plastic).

It takes getting used to. Try to make the transition flow naturally, as if there really is no major change in the way you're eating. You can do this by introducing the changes one at a time. Start with replacing your plate. The others will then come easily.

Your diet may work but you also have to think about what will happen after you exit your program. You would want to be able to at least maintain the weight that you achieved through your diet.

This is where many dieters have failed. And this is where the slow drop in weight is important; the body doesn't over react to the small decrements.

Remember, it's not just about the food. It's the way you approach your food.

Success in dieting, ultimately, requires you to eat healthier.

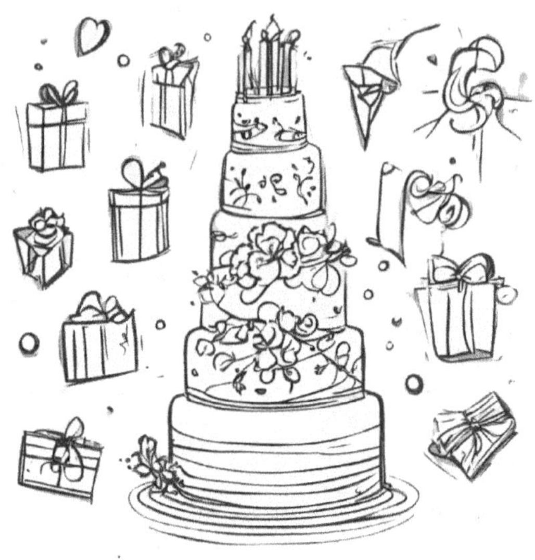

A Special Note for Special Occasions

Imagine this. Your mom just called and she wants you to come over and stay overnight to help her out with your dad's birthday celebration. You know her well of course. Apart from all the guests you have to attend to, she will be attending to feeding you well also. But you're in the middle of a diet.

Or how about this?

You receive a message from a friend who works in another part of the world. You have not seen each other for a long time and she's breezing into town next week. She wants to spend a day with you chatting and visiting new eating places. You really don't have an excuse to refuse, except that you're on a diet.

Or how about this one?

Your cousin is getting married in a few weeks. You guys are quite close, you grew up together. She insists she needs to see you at her wedding and has actually asked you to be her bridesmaid. But you just started your diet and you won't be finished by the time her wedding day rolls around.

And then maybe this.

Your boss has asked you to meet with some business contacts at a high end conference in a hotel. It will be a whole day affair and lunch will be part of it. He's already booked your seat. Are you going to tell him you can't go? You wouldn't want to be rude and not eat because of your diet.

You do have some options. You can call it a cheat day. It is, after all a special occasion. You can probably get back on track in the days that follow.

Or you can just follow the STEPS. Yes, even in a crowd with "forbidden" food all around, the STEPS can help you stay on track.

- **Stop multitasking**. Just focus on one thing at a time. Take some food. If someone tries to engage you in conversation, give a signal that you will respond after you finish chewing what's in your mouth. Then, after you swallow the food, answer the person before you go to your next mouthful. That's just being polite. Remember, don't talk while your mouth is full.

- **Take it slowly**. Chew your food well and don't rush to swallow. It's okay if the person sitting next to you has had two mouthfuls to your one. You'll be digesting your food better and putting off health issues like heartburn and constipation. Besides, you don't want to have critical observers thinking you are a borderline glutton.

- **Enjoy your meal**. Smile and thank the servers. Make it a point to say a good word about the food plating. Talk with the people around you or sitting at the same table. This will also take a little time away from you consuming food. And it makes people think of you as friendly and sociable. That is if you pick the right topics for conversation.

- **Put it down**. Put your utensils down between mouthfuls. Put your cocktail glass down when you go for hors d'oeuvres. Having your hands free may also make communicating with other people easier and will help you avoid accidents like food pieces flying off the fork or your drink spilling on another person. Plus, it will allow for some physical contact with your hands.

- **Size does matter**. Be conscious of your portion and bite sizes. When eating out, you'll probably get a regular sized dinner plate so remember to get less than you usually would. This is especially applicable and actually easier at a buffet. One small piece of fried chicken or half a scoop of something else. At a buffet, you have control of your portion sizes so go ahead and indulge the right way.

So there you go. The STEPS can work anywhere and anytime you eat. You can celebrate with friends and family without putting your diet in jeopardy.

Acknowledgement

I am grateful to a few friends who helped me put this book together.

Let me start with my writing buddies, Paz and Darl with whom the plan was hatched.

Thanks to Jeffrey (IG @jeffreycostales) for half of the illustrations. The rest, I did in Canva.

Thanks to Grace and Paz for the encouraging feedback about the manuscript.

Of course, thank you God for the talent and the opportunity.